THE ALL-INCLUSIVE ANTI-INFLAMMATOR Y DIET

A Stress-Free Meal Plan with 30 Simple Recipes to Strengthen Your Immune System

EMMA Y. TAYLOR

TABLE OF CONTENTS

INTRODUCTION

A STRESS-FREE MEAL PLAN

1. Blueberry Almond Chia Pudding
2. Salmon Avocado Salad
3. Quinoa Stuffed Bell Peppers
4. Turmeric Ginger Carrot Soup
5. Mango Turmeric Smoothie Bowl
6. Cauliflower Rice Stir-Fry
7. Walnut-Crusted Baked Chicken
8. Beetroot and Orange Salad
9. Sweet Potato Lentil Curry
10. Broccoli and Kale Pesto Pasta
11. Chickpea Spinach Curry

12. Asparagus and Lemon Risotto
13. Pomegranate Walnut Chicken Salad
14. Zucchini Noodles with Tomato Basil Sauce
15. Green Bean Almondine
16. Coconut Turmeric Rice
17. Baked Cod with Herbs
18. Brussels Sprouts Quinoa Bowl
19. Lemon Garlic Shrimp Skewers
20. Mushroom Spinach Quiche
21. Sweet Potato Black Bean Chili
22. Avocado Cilantro Lime Rice
23. Roasted Red Pepper Hummus Wrap
24. Cabbage and Apple Slaw
25. Eggplant Tomato Stack
26. Cilantro Lime Shrimp Tacos
27. Raspberry Almond Chia Smoothie
28. Chickpea Avocado Salad
29. Mango Cucumber Salsa:
30. Quinoa Stuffed Acorn Squash

CONCLUSIONS

INTRODUCTION

The Anti-Inflammatory Diet stands as a nutritional approach designed to foster holistic well-being by harnessing the potential of foods recognized for their anti-inflammatory properties. In the contemporary landscape of health and wellness, chronic inflammation has emerged as a key concern, implicated in various ailments such as heart disease, arthritis, and certain types of cancer. The core philosophy of this dietary regimen revolves around cultivating habits that mitigate inflammation within the body.

At the heart of the Anti-Inflammatory Diet lies a commitment to whole foods — an assortment of nutrient-rich, unprocessed ingredients that form the cornerstone of a health-conscious lifestyle. Fruits and vegetables, in their unadulterated forms, take center stage, offering an abundance of essential vitamins, minerals, and antioxidants. These natural components collectively contribute to the reduction of inflammation and bolster the body's ability to heal and function optimally.

An integral aspect of the diet involves the incorporation of omega-3 fatty acids, renowned for their anti-inflammatory properties. Fatty fish like salmon and mackerel, flaxseeds, chia seeds, and walnuts become pivotal players in this nutritional symphony, providing the body with essential fats that contribute to a balanced inflammatory response. The emphasis on a colorful variety of vegetables stems from the understanding that different hues signify distinct phytochemicals and antioxidants, each with its unique anti-inflammatory benefits.

In the realm of fats, the Anti-Inflammatory Diet champions the consumption of healthy fats, exemplified by avocados, olive oil, and nuts. These sources, rich in monounsaturated fats, not only serve as satisfying components of meals but also contribute to the modulation of inflammation. Herbs and spices play a crucial role in adding both flavor and health benefits to the diet. Turmeric, with its active compound curcumin, takes center stage, accompanied by the likes of ginger and garlic, all recognized for their anti-inflammatory prowess.

The selection of proteins in this dietary approach leans towards lean sources. Poultry, fish, legumes, and tofu make appearances as primary protein providers, promoting satiety and muscle health without adding unnecessary inflammatory triggers. Whole grains, such as quinoa, brown rice, and oats, step in as fiber-rich alternatives to refined grains. This not only contributes to overall gut health but also aids in the reduction of inflammation through improved digestion and nutrient absorption.

A critical facet of the Anti-Inflammatory Diet involves the conscious reduction of processed foods and sugars. The modern diet, often laden with highly processed snacks and sugary beverages, is recognized as a potential source of inflammation triggers. By limiting the intake of such items, individuals following this dietary approach seek to create an environment within their bodies that is less susceptible to the chronic inflammatory responses associated with processed foods.

The 8-week meal plan provided here serves as a practical guide for those looking to embark on the journey of adopting an anti-inflammatory lifestyle. The diversity of recipes ensures that every meal is not only nutritionally sound but also a culinary delight. From wholesome breakfast choices to hearty dinner options, each recipe has been crafted to seamlessly integrate into daily life, making the transition to an anti-inflammatory diet both enjoyable and sustainable.

It is crucial to recognize that individual dietary needs may vary, and this plan can be adapted to suit specific preferences, allergies, or health conditions. Before making substantial changes to one's diet, especially for those with pre-existing health concerns, consultation with a healthcare professional is strongly advised. The Anti-Inflammatory Diet is not merely a temporary regimen but rather a philosophy that seeks to foster enduring health and vitality through mindful and deliberate nutritional choices.

A STRESS-FREE MEAL PLAN

1. Blueberry Almond Chia Pudding

- **Ingredients:**
  - Chia seeds
  - Almond milk
  - Blueberries

- **Preparation:**
  - In a bowl, mix 1/4 cup of chia seeds with 1 cup of almond milk.
  - Give everything a good stir, then cover and refrigerate for four or more hours.
  - Before serving, top with a handful of fresh blueberries.

2. Salmon Avocado Salad

- **Ingredients:**
  - Grilled salmon
  - Mixed greens
  - Avocado
  - Olive oil

- Preparation:

- Grill salmon until cooked through, about 4-5 minutes per side.

- In a large bowl, toss mixed greens with diced avocado.

- Flake the grilled salmon over the salad and drizzle with olive oil.

3. Quinoa Stuffed Bell Peppers

- Ingredients:
- Quinoa
- Bell peppers
- Black beans
- Corn

- Preparation:

- Follow the directions on the package to cook the quinoa.

- In a bowl, mix cooked quinoa with black beans and corn.

- Cut bell peppers in half, remove seeds, and stuff with the quinoa mixture. Bake until peppers are tender.

4. Turmeric Ginger Carrot Soup

- Ingredients:
  - Carrots
  - Ginger
  - Turmeric
  - **Vegetable broth**

- Preparation:
  - Peel and chop carrots, then cook them in a pot with ginger and turmeric.
  - Add vegetable broth and simmer until carrots are soft.
  - Blend the mixture until smooth, and season with salt and pepper.

5. Mango Turmeric Smoothie Bowl

- Ingredients:
  - Mango
  - Turmeric
  - Greek yogurt
  - Granola

- Preparation:
  - Blend mango, a pinch of turmeric, and Greek yogurt until smooth.

- Transfer the smoothie into a bowl and sprinkle your preferred granola on top.

6. Cauliflower Rice Stir-Fry

- Ingredients:
  - Cauliflower rice
  - Mixed vegetables
  - Tofu
  - Soy sauce

- Preparation:
  - Grate cauliflower to create rice-sized pieces.
  - Stir-fry cauliflower rice with mixed vegetables and tofu until heated through.
  - Add your preferred stir-fry sauce or soy sauce for seasoning.

7. Walnut-Crusted Baked Chicken

- Ingredients:
  - Chicken breasts
  - Walnuts
  - Herbs

- Preparation:
  - Coat chicken breasts with crushed walnuts and your favorite herbs.

- Bake in the oven until the chicken is cooked through and the coating is golden brown.

8. Beetroot and Orange Salad

- Ingredients:
- Beetroots
- Oranges
- Arugula
- Feta
- Olive oil

- Preparation:
- Roast beetroots until tender, then peel and dice them.
- Toss diced beetroots with orange segments, arugula, and crumbled feta.
- Add a drizzle of olive oil and season with pepper and salt.

9. Sweet Potato Lentil Curry

- Ingredients:
- Sweet potatoes
- Lentils
- Coconut milk
- Curry spices

- Preparation:

- Cook lentils and sweet potatoes in coconut milk until tender.

- Add curry spices and simmer until flavors meld together.

10. Broccoli and Kale Pesto Pasta

- Ingredients:
- Whole-grain pasta
- Broccoli
- Kale
- Pine nuts
- Olive oil

- Preparation:

- Cook whole-grain pasta according to package instructions.

- In a blender, combine steamed broccoli, kale, pine nuts, and a touch of olive oil to make a pesto.

- Serve the cooked pasta by tossing it with the pesto.

11. Chickpea Spinach Curry

- Ingredients:
- Chickpeas
- Spinach

- Tomatoes
- Curry spices

- Preparation:
  - Cook chickpeas with spinach, tomatoes, and curry spices.
  - Simmer until flavors are well combined.

12. Asparagus and Lemon Risotto

- Ingredients:
  - Arborio rice
  - Asparagus
  - Lemon

- Preparation:
  - As directed on the package, prepare the risotto.
  - Stir in cooked asparagus and lemon zest.

13. Pomegranate Walnut Chicken Salad

- Ingredients:
  - Grilled chicken
  - Mixed greens
  - Pomegranate seeds
  - Walnuts

- **Preparation:**
    - Toss mixed greens with grilled chicken, pomegranate seeds, and walnuts.
  - Drizzle with your favorite vinaigrette.

14. Zucchini Noodles with Tomato Basil Sauce

- **Ingredients:**
  - Zucchini noodles
  - Cherry tomatoes
  - Basil

- **Preparation:**
    - Sauté zucchini noodles and toss with cherry tomatoes and basil sauce.

15. Green Bean Almondine

- **Ingredients:**
  - Green beans
  - Almonds
  - Lemon

- **Preparation:**
  - Steam green beans until tender.
  - Sauté with almonds and a squeeze of lemon.

16. Coconut Turmeric Rice

- Ingredients:
- Basmati rice
- Coconut milk
- Turmeric

- Preparation:
  - Cook rice in coconut milk with a pinch of turmeric until fluffy.

17. Baked Cod with Herbs

- Ingredients:
- Cod filets
- Herbs
- Lemon
- Preparation:
  - Coat cod with a mixture of herbs, then bake until flaky.
  - Add a squeeze of fresh lemon on top.

18. Brussels Sprouts Quinoa Bowl

- Ingredients:
- Brussels sprouts
- Quinoa
- Cranberries

- Preparation:

- Roast Brussels sprouts, mix with cooked quinoa and cranberries.

19. Lemon Garlic Shrimp Skewers

- Ingredients:
- Shrimp
- Garlic
- Lemon

- Preparation:

- Marinate shrimp with minced garlic and lemon juice.
- Skewer and grill until cooked.

20. Mushroom Spinach Quiche

- Ingredients:
- Pie crust
- Mushrooms
- Spinach
- Eggs

- Preparation:

- Sauté mushrooms and spinach, then line a pie crust with them.

- Pour beaten eggs over the vegetables and bake until set.

21. Sweet Potato Black Bean Chili

- Ingredients:
- Sweet potatoes
- Black beans
- Tomatoes
- Chili spices

- Preparation:

- Cook sweet potatoes, black beans, and tomatoes with chili spices.

- Simmer until flavors meld together.

22. Avocado Cilantro Lime Rice

- Ingredients:
- Brown rice
- Avocado
- Cilantro
- Lime

- Preparation:

- Mix cooked brown rice with mashed avocado, chopped cilantro, and lime juice.

23. Roasted Red Pepper Hummus Wrap

- Ingredients:
- Whole-grain wrap
- Hummus
- Roasted red peppers

- Preparation:

- Spread hummus on a whole-grain wrap, add roasted red peppers, and roll.

24. Cabbage and Apple Slaw

- Ingredients:
- Green cabbage
- Apples
- Greek yogurt dressing
- Preparation:

- Shred green cabbage, mix with sliced apples, and toss with Greek yogurt dressing.

25. Eggplant Tomato Stack

- Ingredients:
- Eggplant
- Tomatoes
- Mozzarella

- Preparation:
- Grill or roast eggplant and tomato slices.
- Stack them with mozzarella and drizzle with balsamic.

26. Cilantro Lime Shrimp Tacos

- Ingredients:
- Shrimp
- Corn tortillas
- Cilantro
- Lime

- Preparation:
- Sauté shrimp with chopped cilantro and lime.
- Fill corn tortillas with the shrimp mixture.

# 27.	Raspberry	Almond	Chia Smoothie

- Ingredients:
- Almond milk
- Raspberries
- Chia seeds

- Preparation:
- Blend almond milk, raspberries, and chia seeds until smooth.

28. Chickpea Avocado Salad

- Ingredients:
- Chickpeas
- Avocado
- Cherry tomatoes

- Preparation:
- **Mix chickpeas,** diced avocado, and halved cherry tomatoes.
- Add a drizzle of olive oil and season with pepper and salt.

29. Mango Cucumber Salsa:

- Ingredients:

- Mango
- Cucumber
- Red onion
- Lime

- Preparation:
- Chop the red onion, cucumber, and mango.
- Toss with freshly squeezed lime juice.

30. Quinoa Stuffed Acorn Squash

- Ingredients:
- Quinoa
- Acorn squash
- Pecans

- Preparation:
- Cook quinoa, stuffed acorn squash halves, and top with chopped pecans.

CONCLUSIONS

In summary, the Anti-Inflammatory Diet positions itself as a comprehensive nutritional strategy that aims to promote general health and wellbeing in addition to reducing inflammation. This dietary philosophy's tenets go beyond a simple set of guidelines; they represent a significant movement toward the acceptance of nutrient-dense, whole foods as the cornerstone of a healthful way of life.

With processed and convenience foods frequently taking center stage in our dietary landscape, the Anti-Inflammatory Diet becomes increasingly important as we navigate the complexities of modern living. It challenges us to reconsider the foods we eat, emphasizing foods that support the body's defense mechanism against chronic inflammation. This diet provides a path to a more robust and energetic life by combining a variety of colorful vegetables, lean proteins, healthy fats, and anti-inflammatory herbs and spices.

This 8-week meal plan is more than just a collection of recipes; it's a thoughtful selection meant to make the transition to an anti-inflammatory lifestyle approachable and pleasurable. The variety and depth of the dishes offer a real-world example of how applying these ideas to our everyday existence may be a delightful and fulfilling experience. Each meal serves as evidence that making healthy food choices doesn't have to sacrifice flavor or enjoyment, from breakfast options that provide energy to supper options that round off a mindful eating day.

That being said, it's critical to approach the Anti-Inflammatory Diet uniquely. The way that each person's body reacts to dietary modifications depends on a variety of factors, including heredity, pre-existing medical issues, and personal preferences. Because of this, the meal plan is a flexible guidance that may be adjusted to suit individual requirements and circumstances rather than a strict prescription.

Consulting a healthcare provider before making any major dietary changes is a wise course of action. They are able to provide tailored guidance by considering each person's unique health profile and any sensitivities. Fundamentally, the Anti-Inflammatory Diet is a way of life, and its advantages go well beyond the short-term reduction of inflammation. It's a dedication to long-term health, lifespan promotion, and cultivating an intentional and aware connection with food.

Within the dynamic field of nutritional research, the Anti-Inflammatory Diet serves as a guiding principle for rational and scientifically supported dietary practices. This nutritional approach challenges us to view food not just as subsistence but as a powerful instrument for fostering resilience and vigor as we work toward healthier and more fulfilled lives. By following the Anti-Inflammatory Diet's guidelines, we set out on a path to a more energetic and nourished life in which each meal serves as a chance to improve and maintain our general health.